Mikkael Duarte dos Santos
J. Péricles M. Vasconcelos

Short bowel syndrome

AF294272

Mikkael Duarte dos Santos
J. Péricles M. Vasconcelos

Short bowel syndrome

Clinical and surgical management

ScienciaScripts

Imprint

Any brand names and product names mentioned in this book are subject to trademark, brand or patent protection and are trademarks or registered trademarks of their respective holders. The use of brand names, product names, common names, trade names, product descriptions etc. even without a particular marking in this work is in no way to be construed to mean that such names may be regarded as unrestricted in respect of trademark and brand protection legislation and could thus be used by anyone.

Cover image: www.ingimage.com

This book is a translation from the original published under ISBN 978-613-9-72065-1.

Publisher:
Sciencia Scripts
is a trademark of
Dodo Books Indian Ocean Ltd. and OmniScriptum S.R.L publishing group

120 High Road, East Finchley, London, N2 9ED, United Kingdom
Str. Armeneasca 28/1, office 1, Chisinau MD-2012, Republic of Moldova, Europe
Printed at: see last page
ISBN: 978-620-7-72634-9

Copyright © Mikkael Duarte dos Santos, J. Péricles M. Vasconcelos
Copyright © 2024 Dodo Books Indian Ocean Ltd. and OmniScriptum S.R.L publishing group

To the man who lived more than a hundred
years in just over two decades and taught
(and practised) the full concept of life:
Rembrandt F. R. M. da Rocha *(in
memorian).*

ACKNOWLEDGEMENTS

A single page of a monograph, no matter how labour-intensive and exhaustive it may have been, does not illustrate, even in a tiny way, the infinite gratitude I have for all the people who have been with me over the last twenty-three years of my life.

To my father, Manoel P. dos Santos and my mother, Marleide Mª D. dos Santos, for their support (in every way).

To my siblings, Marcos, Nyelson and Michelly, as well as to my family for existing.

To my girlfriend, Tamiris, for putting up with me and loving me despite my misadventures and unstable moods.

To my endless list of great friends: Beethoven, Belize, Carlos, Danúzio, George, Heli, Joao Adolfo, Joel, Jonatas, José N. de Alencar, Juan, Luís Rufino, Luiz Halley, Mário, Roberta, Shirley, Tarsízio and Wendson. I am who you moulded me to be.

To Mrs Damiana de Sousa Leite *(in memorian),* my patient, for trusting me so much and for inspiring me to do this work. May it help to change the fate of others who suffer as she did.

To Walden, master of the art of understanding the complete composition of everything, for teaching me a pinch of his knowledge.

If I knew before what I know now, I'd get everything exactly wrong...

Humberto Gessinger

SUMMARY

Short bowel syndrome (SIS) is characterised by intestinal insufficiency, most often the result of extensive intestinal resection; it causes severe hydroelectrolytic and nutritional disorders such as vitamin deficiency and malnutrition. The primary objectives of this book are to explain and analyse the various forms of clinical and surgical management, both traditional and innovative. Through a systematic review of the literature, it attempts to examine the most recent studies (case reports, clinical trials, textbooks and articles of general scientific relevance) published in English, Spanish and Portuguese on short bowel syndrome - primarily in the last ten years. In recent times, greater clarity about the pathophysiological and adaptive mechanisms that occur in the short intestine has led to progress in surgical techniques, new drugs and the promising technique of intestinal tissue engineering, thus promoting greater expectations and expectations among health professionals and, above all, among those suffering from this syndrome. This study shows that parenteral nutrition is still indispensable in the management of patients with CIS, but it has enormous limitations due to its prolonged use, including its cost, infections associated with the catheter and liver disease associated with parenteral nutrition. There are numerous studies suggesting that a new era of clinical treatment is approaching, involving drugs such as GLP-2, GH, teduglutide, EGF, IGF-1 and glu- tamine stimulating development and encouraging greater absorption of the remaining intestine; unfortunately, for the time being, research in humans is scarce. Intestinal transplantation still presents barriers today, especially with regard to graft rejection. Various non-transplant surgical techniques have been described around the world in an attempt to palliate and become alternatives to transplantation (a therapeutic modality available in only a few centres). The high morbidity and mortality of this clinical condition is striking and several studies are still needed to reach a consensus on its treatment.

Keywords: Short bowel syndrome. Intestinal transplantation. Parenteral nutrition

SUMMARY

1 INTRODUCTION

Short bowel syndrome (SBS) is a clinical condition that encompasses numerous concepts. Some authors argue that the definition of SBS refers predominantly to the length and magnitude of the bowel resection. For Castillo et al. (1996) SCI is characterised "as a functional length of the small intestine distal to the Treitz angle of less than 50% of the expected normal". Intestinal length in humans is not a constant; it depends *in vivo on* muscle tone, as well as anatomical variants. In general, measured from the duodenal-jejunal flexure, the length of the intestine varies between 275 cm and 850 cm (PEN- NINGTON et al., 2003). Joly et al. (2009) describe the syndrome in adults as a functioning intestine of less than 200 cm.

In fact, what most authors corroborate is the concept that IBS denotes a circumstance, independent of the absolute length of the intestine, where intestinal function is compromised. This is how Chagas Neto et al. (2011) conceptualise it: "SCI is defined by the inability of the surface of the small intestine to maintain adequate conditions for nutrient absorption, causing nutritional deficiencies."

The prevalence of CIS is as high as 4 per million inhabitants. According to Cole et al. (2008) it affects 2,200 US adults and children. Intestinal failure due to CIS occurs in up to 15 per cent of patients who undergo intestinal resection (DIBIASE, J.K; YOUNG, R.J; VANDERHOOF, J.A., 2004). Roughly speaking, without taking into account factors that directly or indirectly interfere with the survival of patients with CIS, we can see that around 70 per cent of these patients remain alive within a year (SEETHARAM, P.; RODRIGUES G., 2011). Spencer et al. (2008) report that the cost, between home and hospital care, can reach 250000 thousand dollars/year.

In the paediatric population, as in adults, CIS is the biggest cause of intestinal failure. The neonatal age group accounts for 80 per cent of the syndrome's cases; although

Despite the extremely high morbidity, 80% of these neonates survive in the long term (MARTINEZ et al., 2011). Spencer et al. (2005) suggest that for CIS survival in infants and children, at least 15 cm with an intact ileo-cecal valve (ICV) or 40 cm without an ICV is required.

CIS presents health professionals (doctors, nutritionists, psychologists, nurses...) and any researcher trying to explore the subject with a huge challenge.

On the one hand, when conservative therapy is chosen, the dichotomy comes into play: enteral nutrition (EN) versus parenteral nutrition (PN). It is well known that patients with CIS who use only PN have impaired intestinal adaptation after resection, to the detriment of those who use PN, prolonging the need for the former in a vicious cycle (SEETHARAM, P.; RODRIGUES G., 2011). However, the evolution of CIS in the pre-NP era held a sombre prognosis for its patients (SPENCER et al., 2005), which shows us the great relevance of NP in patients with intestinal insufficiency.

When it comes to surgical treatment, some fundamental aspects must be considered if the chosen technique is to be successful. The primary objective of surgical therapy, which is to increase the functional capacity of the intestine, must guide the surgeon's behaviour. The attempt to preserve the existing intestine is the fundamental pillar if the patient's survival is not to be unsuccessful. In general, the techniques used today try to improve bowel function, motility and prolong intestinal transit. Bowel transplantation is still a growing therapeutic modality, but one that poses major challenges for the medical team (SEETHARAM, P.; RODRIGUES G., 2011).

In view of the above, we are forced to navigate an ocean of questions (still with imprecise answers) about how to manage a patient with CIS. To what extent should we use PN as opposed to costs, side effects and a deficit in intestinal readaptation? When (and how) should we introduce NE? What patients will the benefits of surgical therapy (including transplantation) outweigh its costs?

This work is justified in view of the difficulties that doctors and the healthcare team have in examining and scrutinising these questions in order to overcome the challenges that the management, whether clinical or surgical, of patients with CIS imposes.

2 OBJECTIVES

2.1 General

A nalyse the various forms of clinical and surgical management of CIS.

2.2 Specific

Evidence of the aetiology and pathophysiology, as well as complications of CIS.

Explain the cost-benefit of parenteral and enteral nutrition.

Demonstrate the advantages and disadvantages of new and old drugs in the management of CIS.

Follow the evolution of the various surgical techniques in recent years.

Discuss new surgical management modalities for CIS.

3 METHODOLOGY

3.1 Study design

In view of the objectives set out above, we classify this work as exploratory research of the literature review type, with a qualitative approach. Exploratory research aims to provide greater familiarity with the problem, with a view to making it more explicit or forming hypotheses (GIL, 2002).

Literature review research is carried out on the basis of the available record of a given topic. "The texts become sources of the themes to be researched". Its aim is to put the researcher in touch with what has been written previously on a given subject (MARCONI; LAKATOS, 2005; SEVERINO, 2007).

Qualitative research arises from the impossibility of investigating and understanding some phenomena that focus on perception, intuition and subjectivity using statistical data. Despite being recognised by academics, the term 'qualitative research' or even 'qualitative methodology' does not specifically refer to a type of research. "That's why it's preferable to talk about [...] qualitative approaches, as these names refer to sets of methodologies." (SEVERINO, 2007).

3.2 The process of acquiring literature

3.2.1 Study period

The sources selected for this study primarily comprise articles from the last ten years, given the current nature of these sources. Bibliographical sources from the last few decades are also used, as they are considered "classics" and are routinely used in more current articles.

3.2.2 Database

Articles were extracted from scientific article collection sites such as *PUBMED, HIGHWIRE, SCIELO, LILACS and BIBLIOTECA CONCHRANE, as* well as books and conference proceedings on the subject.

3.2.3 Study inclusion criteria

Texts, books, annals and scientific articles that contain information that can elucidate the questions that guide this research are used. Exploratory studies such as literature reviews and descriptive studies in Portuguese, English and Spanish are used.

1.1 Ethical aspects

The texts used as a basis for the review are only scientific in nature and will deal, either directly or indirectly, with the topic to be dealt with in this project, respecting any aspect of the publications' copyright.

4 LITERATURE REVIEW

4.1 Etiology

Undoubtedly, the main cause of CIS in both the adult and paediatric populations is the loss of bowel function due to extensive resection (HASOSAH et al., 2008). The reasons that lead to this resection differ between age groups.

In adults, the reasons for CIS are diverse: Crohn's disease, mesenteric ischaemia, trauma, volvulus, radiation enteritis, among others (WANG et al., 2007). Table 1.

Table 1 - Most common causes of CIS

ADULTS	NEONATES
- Crohn's disease	- Necrotising enteritis
- Mesenteric ischaemia	- Atresia of the small intestine
• Surgical procedures for malig- nity and trauma	• Intestinal malrotation
• Radiation enteritis	• Volvo
• Jejuno-ileal diversion for obesity	

Source: (BANERJEE; WARWICKER, 2002, p. 38).

Among paediatric cases, neonates account for the majority: around 80% (MARTINEZ et al., 2011). Of these, the absolute majority of intestinal resections are caused by necrotising enterocolitis (96%), followed by congenital malformations (intestinal atresia and gastroschisis) and intestinal volvulus (2% each) (COLE et al., 2008). Table 1.

In very rare cases, CIS can be congenital. Only 37 cases of congenital SCI have been described in the English literature. Theories have been proposed to justify the origin of this condition, such as ischaemia, which is usually secondary to necrotising enterocolitis, causing intestinal infarction; defective intra-uterine neurodevelopment or even abnormalities in the myenteric plexus. However, the exact cause and aetiopathogenesis of congenital CIS are not fully understood (PALLE, L.; REDDY, B., 2010). Some reports have associated congenital SCI with anomalies such as pyloric stenosis, agenesis of the appendix and dextrocardia (HASOSAH et al., 2008).

1.2 Pathophysiology

The main consequence of extensive intestinal resection is the loss of absorption surface area, which results in malabsorption of macro and micronutrients, electrolytes and water, which has the clinical effect of voluminous diarrhoea, hypovolaemia, hypo-natremia and hypokalaemia.

Most macronutrients are absorbed in the proximal 100-150 cm of the intestine, while micronutrient absorption is restricted to certain areas of the small intestine. Phosphorus, iron and water-soluble vitamins are predominantly absorbed in the proximal small intestine; as most patients with CIS have an intact duodenum and proximal jejunum, deficiencies of these entities are rare, but they tend to develop calcium and magnesium deficiencies. The loss of part or all of the ileum will result in malabsorption of vitamin B12 and salts (GARCIA, M.M; ME- NENDEZ-CONDE, C.P.; VICEDO, T.B, 2011; SEETHARAM, P.; RODRIGUES G., 2011).

If the remaining intestine is longer than 100cm, there is a good chance that these patients will tolerate oral feeding for a short period of time. If the length is between 50 and 100 cm, the patient will need NP for a short period of time and will probably continue regular oral nutrition on their own. Patients with an intestine shorter than 50 cm will generally develop permanent intestinal insufficiency (KEMP et al., 2006).

However, although the remaining length of the intestine is a determining factor in the condition of a patient with CIS, the reduction in the absorptive capacity of the intestine after major resections is not just a reflection of the reduction in intestinal length - several other components contribute. Intestinal resection is followed by hypersecretion of gastric acid due to the loss of inhibitory peptides. Not only does the acidic environment impair digestion through its effect on the pancreas and other digestive enzymes, but the precipitation of bile acids increases the problem of lipid malabsorption. Similarly, the loss of peptides such as glucagon-like peptide 2 (GLP- 2) and peptide YY, resulting from ileal loss, causes an acceleration in gastric emptying and intestinal transit. Thus, gastric hypersecretion, impaired digestion and rapid intestinal transit combine to reduce the residual function of the intestine (PENNINGTON et al., 2003). In CIS, the status of gastrin, cholecystokinin, secretin, gastric inhibitory polypeptide and motilin, which are produced by endocrine cells in the proximal gastrointestinal tract, remains intact (SEETHA- RAM, P.; RODRIGUES G., 2011).

There is also an increase in the incidence of cholelithiasis - probably due to gallbladder stasis and the breakdown of the enterohepatic circulation. The number of symptomatic nephrolithiasis has increased. Malabsorption of fats, inducing bile salts to increase the absorption of oxalate by the colon, hyperoxaluria, as well as a reduction in bacterial degradation explain the genesis of kidney stones (NIGHTINGALE J.; WOODWARD M., 2006; TOWSEND et al., 2005).

The presence of the ileocecal junction improves the functional capacity of the intestinal remnant and its subsequent adaptation, as we will see below (SEETHARAM, P.; RODRIGUES G., 2011).

1.2.1 Intestinal adaptation

Intestinal adaptation is defined as what happens after intestinal loss, whether it is progressive recovery from intestinal insufficiency or failure to recover (JEPPESEN et al., 2003).

Several examples of adaptation in animal models have already been described: chronic ethanol ingestion, sublethal doses of abdominal irradiation, diabetes, ageing, fasting and malnutrition. However, due to the existence of various relevant anatomical, physiological and biochemical differences between the animals studied and the gastrointestinal tract (as well as an obvious lack of comparable studies in humans), the true clinical correlation between the animal models researched and the adaptation that occurs in humans remains to be determined; therefore, it is not yet known exactly how this adaptation occurs in human intestines (DROZDOWSKI, L., THOMSON, A.B.R., 2006).

What is known, however, is that as time passes, the remaining part of the parched intestine tries to adapt by thickening, hyperplasia, as well as dilation of its wall and decreased motility. These morpho-physiological changes result in an increase in intestinal transit time and, consequently, improve absorption, a condition that tends to alleviate the clinical condition (NONINO etal., 2001).

Intestinal adaptation mechanisms occur at various levels: physiological, cellular and molecular. These mechanisms tend to be different depending on the location (the ileum has a greater capacity for adaptation than the jejunum), the region of the tissue (crypts or ends of the villi) and the extent of the intestinal resection (the greater the intestinal resection, the greater the attempt at adaptation), which would explain the fact that there are site-specific alterations and differences between enterocytes (GUPTE et al., 2006). The presence or absence of the ileocecal valve, location (jejunum versus ileum, age of the patient and comorbidities such as underlying disease like Crohn's, radiation enteritis, carcinoma and pseudo-obstruction) are also variants that influence the adaptation process and clinical evolution (KEMP et al., 2006).

In addition to these factors already mentioned, we include gastrointestinal regulatory peptides, growth factors, hormones, cytokines and tissue factors that include immunity, blood flow and neural influences as relevant in adaptation.
(SEETHARAM, P.; RODRIGUES G., 2011).

Didactically, we will divide these adaptive processes temporally:

> [...] They occur in three distinct periods in the post-operative period. In the first, which lasts up to 3 months, there is a hydro-electrolytic imbalance due to intense diarrhoea. In this phase, nutrition must be provided exclusively via the parenteral route, with the concomitant replacement of fluids and electrolytes being of fundamental importance. The second stage, lasting up to a year, corresponds to the adaptation period in which the diarrhoea stabilises, allowing the oral diet to begin. In the third stage, maximum adaptation is achieved and the oral diet is prepared in such a way as to offer all the nutrients needed to maintain a good nutritional state (NONINO et al., 2001, p. 202).

The insufficient intestine can also go through a number of possibilities during its adaptation process, and these possibilities are subject to the existence or not of therapeutic intervention. Figure 1 shows these theoretical possibilities of adaptation that the post-resection gut can follow.

'Spontaneous adaptation' of intestinal function is that which generally evolves idiosyncratically, without any kind of intervention, towards a plateau of adaptation

(JEPPESEN et al., 2003).

When trying to improve intestinal adaptation, some therapies (discussed below) can cause adaptation to reach a high plateau phase ('Accelerated Hyperadaptation' and 'Hyperadaptation'), or reduce the length of time until the plateau is reached ('Accelerated Adaptation'). (JEPPESEN et al., 2003).

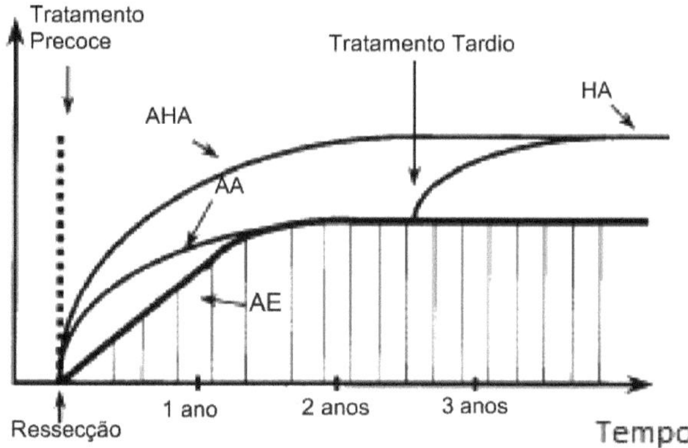

Figure 1 Scheme of intestinal adaptation
LEGEND: AE, spontaneous adaptation; AA, accelerated adaptation; HA, hyper-adaptation; AHA, accelerated hyper-adaptation.
SOURCE: Jeppesen et al. (2003, p. 3722).

1.3 Clinical picture and complications

We can divide the clinical picture of a patient with CIS according to the intestinal adaptive phase and correlate it with the symptoms they manifest. Clinically, it is generally characterised by chronic diarrhoea, dehydration, electrolyte disorders and nutritional deficits with progressive malnutrition (PAREKH, N.; SEIDNER D.; STEIGER E., 2005; WU et al., 2003).

The acute phase begins in the immediate post-operative period and lasts for the first few months. As a result of gastric hypersecretion, the great loss of absorptive capacity and increased intestinal motility, severe diarrhoea and steatorrhoea remain the main clinical manifestations of CIS. (SAFIOLEAS et al., 2008).

In this phase, water loss, due to intense diarrhoea (5 to 20 times a day), worsens with oral intake and can reach 10 litres a day. Severe weight loss is also found in the acute phase, as well as electrolyte disturbances: hypopotassemia, hyponatremia, hypocalcaemia and hypomagnesemia (DANI, 2006). In patients with colon integrity, dehydration or sodium deficiency are rare (NIGHTINGALE J.; WOODWARD M., 2006). Hypomagnesemia is less severe in patients who still have a functioning colon; however, they rarely do not have magnesium depletion (MIRANDA et al., 2000).

After the first few months, the adaptive phase follows, lasting until the second year after resection. The diarrhoea tends to regress and clinically stabilise. The patient already recognises foods that aggravate diarrhoea and therefore modifies their diet. Due to continuous gastric hypersecretion, gastroduodenal lesions deepen (DANI, 2006).

And finally, the chronic phase, where there is a state of clinical and adaptive equilibrium. Weight loss is irreversible; the number of bowel movements is stable (between 2 and 4 times a day), but still with a bulky, pasty appearance (DANI, 2006).

At this stage, complications such as cholelithiasis and nephrolithiasis become common. In up to 45 per cent of patients (the majority male) gallstones are present. A quarter develop symptomatic calcium oxalate nephrolithiasis (NIGHTINGALE J.; WOODWARD M., 2006).

1.4 Clinical management

1.4.1 Initial handling

The main objective (and greatest challenge) of treatment and care for patients with intestinal failure is the rehabilitation of the remaining intestine. Full NS should be the goal; the approach (which should be multidisciplinary) should encompass nutritional measures, pharmacological measures and surgical interventions (LE et al., 2010).

The most important aspect that should guide the doctor who treats a patient with CIS is its prevention:

> In patients with Crohn's disease, resections limited to the particular complication should be performed. In addition, during the operation for problems related to intestinal ischaemia, the smallest possible resection should be performed, and, if necessary, operations should be performed for a second visualisation to allow the ischaemic bowel to be demarcated, thus potentially preventing an unnecessarily extensive resection of the bowel. (TOWSEND et al., 2005, p. 1373).

Special attention should be paid to the post-operative period. There are three pillars that underpin the management of patients with CIS in the early treatment phase: diarrhoea control, fluid replacement and the introduction of NP. (TOWSEND et al., 2005).

Intense diarrhoea can lead to immense hydro-electrolytic losses, resulting in severe dehydration, hypotension and pre-renal insufficiency. Periodic assessment of the patient should initially be carried out every 1-2 days, then once or twice a week and, in the long term, at least every three months. This assessment should always include electrolyte and nitrogen slag levels, as well as anthropometric measurements (weight, BMI, percentage weight loss and circular arm circumference) (NIGHTINGALE J.; WOODWARD M., 2006).

Some drugs are helpful in controlling steatorrhoea and diarrhoea. Antidiarrhoeals are almost always useful. The most commonly used: loperamide, diphenoxylate, codeine and antiemetics should be taken thirty minutes to one hour before each meal and at bedtime (PAREKH, N.; SEIDNER D.; STEIGER E., 2005). Octreotide, a somatostatin analogue, in the acute phase, by reducing gastric hypersecretion, also seems to have an influence on reducing diarrhoea (TOWSEND et al., 2005). Bile acid resins, such as cholestyramine, have been reported as a good choice for anti-diarrhoea therapy in patients who have an intact colon and voluminous bowel movements due to loss of bile salts; a major drawback of this treatment is that cholestyramine can cause or aggravate steatorrhoea in patients who have had a more massive ileal resection (with a residual intestine smaller than 100cm) or who do not have an intact colon. (SEETHARAM, P.; RODRIGUES G., 2011).

An important point to emphasise in the early management of patients with intestinal insufficiency due to CIS is the immediate introduction of proton pump inhibitors or H2 blockers; these patients (who are hypergastrinemic) are extremely susceptible to ulcerations in the gastrointestinal tract over the course of a few months, and should at least use these medications (in moderate to high doses) in the first three to six months after resection (PAREKH, N.; SEIDNER D.; STEIGER E., 2005). Treatment with these drugs also helps to improve diarrhoea, given that gastric hypersecretion is part of the pathophysiological spectrum of this condition in CIS. (TOWSEND et al., 2005).

The first three weeks are characterised by a disturbance in water and electrolyte homeostasis. Patients with CIS have an increased demand for fluids and electrolytes during this period, due to the large amount lost through faeces and the nasogastric tube, and therefore require sparing intravenous replacement. This infusion (which covers sensitive and insensitive losses) should gradually be replaced by oral intake (DANI, 2006).

A specific problem is lactic acidosis, which results from the bacterial fermentation of nutrients (particularly simple sugars) that are not absorbed. Diagnosis is suggested by unexplained metabolic acidosis and associated neurological symptoms. Treatment includes minimising total calorie intake or instituting a low-carbohydrate diet. The administration of intestinal-spectrum antibiotics, such as metronidazole, may be appropriate (SEETHARAM, P.; RODRIGUES G., 2011).

NP is extremely important in the immediate post-operative period: it provides a great prognostic improvement in patients with CIS, but in addition to the high costs, it reserves long-term risks. The use of NP will be discussed in more detail below.

1.4.2 Nutritional Management

4.4.2.1 *Parenteral nutrition*

The NIDDKD (National Institute of Diabetes and Digestive and Kidney Diseases) stated that in 2002 alone, twenty thousand patients used PN in the United States (GURA et al., 2008). The first report of parenteral use for human nutrition dates back to the late 1960s. Greater survival was achieved in subsequent years in neonates with congenital short bowel (the first patients to use PN) who used this new form of nutrition (TANNURI, 2004).

CIS is one of the main indications for the use of NP; its use is well founded for the prevention of severe malnutrition in patients who have intestinal insufficiency, i.e. are unable to absorb nutrients administered orally or enterally (DURAN, 2005). Not using PN is associated with a six-month survival rate in patients who have undergone intestinal resection of more than two metres (UNAMUNO et al., 2005).

Immediate use of NP is essential in patients undergoing massive intestinal resection; its early use is associated with improved prognosis and increased survival (COLE et al., 2010). Total NP should be maintained for at least the first 10 to 70 postoperative days. According to the American Gastroenterological Association (AGA), until clinical stability is achieved, NP cannot be withdrawn (DURAN, 2005).

The duration of exclusive use of NP is directly related to the remaining length of the intestine. In addition to length, the amount of energy and protein provided by NP, the use and tolerability of NP, age, weight and height of the patient all contribute to successful weaning from NP (BORGES et al., 2011).

Despite the aforementioned advantages, the long-term use of NP, besides being immensely expensive financially, carries with it many mechanical, infectious and metabolic complications that test its real benefit against its cost (BORGES et al., 2011).

Technical (mechanical) complications are generally related to the placement of the catheter: catheter thrombosis, haemothorax, pneumothorax, etc. An early sign of catheter thrombosis is slow or no blood return to the catheter under aspiration. Effective treatment to dissolve the thrombus is thrombolytic therapy (DURAN, 2005).

Catheter-related infections are the most common complications, with an incidence of around 3 to 20 per cent (directly proportional to the severity of the case). The most commonly implicated agent is coagulase-negative *staphylococcus* (multi-resistant *Staphylococcus epidermis*). *Staphylococus aureus,* fungi and gram-negative bacilli are also common. These infections are difficult to diagnose and treat because they are caused by hospital germs; therefore, the prevention of infection through catheter care by healthcare professionals is of fundamental importance (UNA- MUNO et al., 2005).

Two measures, still under study, can be tried to prevent catheter infection. The first refers to the use of antibiotics such as vancomycin, cipro- floxacin, gentamicin and amphotericin B; this measure has achieved efficacy ranging from 30 to 100 per cent. The second measure is the use of ethanol locks. This approach does not induce bacterial resistance. By denaturing proteins, ethanol is rapidly bactericidal and fungicidal (LE et al.,

2010).

The use of antibiotic-coated catheters has also been studied in an effort to reduce the rate of central catheter infections. They are not widely accepted due to their high cost. However, catheters coated with minocycline and rifampicin have been shown to be effective in delaying the onset of infection without increasing the risk of thrombosis (Le et al., 2010).

NP is also linked to an increased incidence of infections in general, as it is imbricated with a deficit in mucosal immunity, increased intestinal permeability, bacterial overgrowth and translocation, impaired neutrophil function and atrophy of the mucosal architectonics (DURAN, 2005). In animal models, NE, unlike NP, has been linked to increased intestinal mucosal immunity (COLE et al., 2010).

Duran (2005) suggests that lipid emulsions administered in PN impair the bactericidal and migratory functions of PMN (polymorphonuclear cells) and cause phagocyte dysfunction, resulting in greater susceptibility to infections (bacteraemia, pneumonia and abscesses). Long-chain triglycerides (lipid components of PN) have an immunosuppressive effect by interfering with the binding of interleukin 2 (IL-2).

At the start of NP infusion, glucose intolerance is the main adverse effect; therefore, a minimum of four daily glucose checks should be carried out. The glycaemic level should not exceed 180-200 mg/dl (DURAN, 2005).

These complications are associated with increased morbidity and mortality. Messing (1999 apud BORGES et al., 2011) carried out a study of 124 patients with SCI and found a 10-year mortality rate of 53 per cent. Death was related to NP use and complications in 22 per cent of cases.

Some of these complications can be minimised or even remedied through the technique of administering PN in cycles (Parenteral Nutrition Cycling). In short, NP cycling is defined as giving the entire daily volume of NP in less than 24 hours. Inherent in the method are the advantages of disconnecting the central access (which vitally reduces the risk of infection, bacteraemia and sepsis) and reducing the incidence of hyperinsulinaemia (LE et al., 2010).

The NP cycling procedure is indicated for patients who will be using NP for a long time (more than 30 days) and who have balanced cardiac, renal and endocrine function and can tolerate relatively wide glycaemic variations. The patient must be metabolically stable for several days before attempting this technique. There is a risk of marked changes in glycaemia; to avoid such risks, the infusion rate of the parenteral solution should be gradually increased in the first two hours and slowly decreased in the last hour (LE et al., 2010).

Another measure pointed out as effective by Borges et al. (2011) to reduce the deleterious consequences of prolonged use of NP is its intermittent use throughout the year. It should be considered as a nutritional 'aid' for patients who are not adequately nourished by oral intake alone.

A major cost of the prolonged use of NP is recurrent hospital admissions and the associated harm (increased risk of multi-resistant infection, increased costs, as well as the closely associated psychological damage). Tannuri (2004) carried out a retrospective study of 19 children with CIS who required long-term PN (8 months to 4 years in the study), which found:

> Every child admitted to hospital with the prospect of prolonged intravenous nutritional treatment should be considered for direct transfer to their home, after the initial period of stabilisation of clinical conditions. [...] home parenteral nutrition is sometimes the only therapeutic option for children with SCI and promotes a maximum level of comfort for the patient and parents. (TANNURI, 2004, p. 334).

Home NP can be an alternative for patients whose remaining intestine is in the process of adapting and who cannot tolerate oral nutrition. This measure is associated with greater convenience and shorter hospital stays (TANNURI, 2004).

4.4.2.1.1 Parenteral nutrition-associated liver dysfunction (PNALD)

Among the complications linked to PN, Parenteral Nutrition Associated Liver Disease (PNALD) is the most important. The aetiology of this condition is not known for certain; however, it is likely that its genesis is multifactorial. It is characterised by liver dysfunction, ranging from elevated transaminases to liver failure (LE et al., 2010). Table 2 lists the main hepato-biliary alterations linked to NP.

PNALD has a mortality rate of close to 100 per cent in one year in those who are unable to withstand weaning from NP or who have not undergone liver transplantation

(GURA et al., 2006). It is most commonly found in children (especially premature infants) and manifests itself particularly as cholestasis, while in adults it takes on the appearance of steatohepatitis. The prevalence of this clinical condition is unknown, although some studies point to some hepatic alteration in 20 to 90 per cent of patients receiving PN (VILLARES, 2008).

Table 2 - Hepato-biliary complications associated with the use of parenteral nutrition
Source: (VILLARES, 2008, p. 26).

LIVER CHANGES	BILIARY CHANGES
- Steatosis	- Cholestasis
- Steatohepatitis	- Acalculous cholecystitis
- Fibrosis	- Bile sludge
- Cirrhosis	- Cholelithiasis

Villares (2008) divides the risk factors for the development of PNALD into three groups: 1- derived from defective intestinal function as a result of a lack of enteral stimulation; 2- liver toxicants present in PN or the absence of certain nutrients, which would lead to liver damage; and 3- underlying disease.

Frequent surgical procedures, lack of enteral intake, sepsis, prolonged use of PN and prematurity (in congenital or neonatal SCI) are some of the risk factors for developing PNALD. (GURA et al., 2008). As well as sepsis, recurrent infections (the probable source of which is bacterial translocation from the catheter due to permeability or intestinal bacterial overgrowth) are correlated in 30% of cases with the development of PNALD; hence the prevention of catheter-related infection must be given vital importance (LE et al., 2010).

When NP is used for short periods, liver involvement is limited to a small increase in transaminases and its function remains intact. However, when direct bilirubin rises (>2 mg/dl) over a long period of NP use, the first propaedeutic step should be to rule out other causes of liver damage and try to minimise risk factors (VILLARES, 2008).

In the first two weeks of NP use, cholestasis first appears as an increase in gamma GT and alkaline phosphatase, followed later by an increase in bilirubin and transaminases. Kemp et al. (2006) warn that jaundice is a late sign of PNALD. The natural history of this pathology leads to liver cirrhosis, a condition that requires liver and intestinal transplantation (VILLARES, 2008).

Although the aetiology of this clinical condition is unknown, it is believed that the lipid emulsions in NP play a large part. These emulsions, which are derived from soya or sunflower oil, are rich in fatty acids. Attempts have been made to integrate (or replace traditional lipid emulsions) fish oil emulsions into NP, due to their anti-inflammatory and anti-aggregation effects. What has been observed is that omega-3 (the main component of fish oil), through as yet unknown pathways, reduces lipogenesis and prevents or attenuates NP-induced hepatic steatosis (GURA et al., 2006).

Gura et al. (2008) in a cohort study of 18 neonates who depended on PN observed that the use of fish oil-based emulsion was able to reverse cholestasis and fatal liver disease, which resulted in the absence of liver transplants in these children.

Borges et al. (2011) cite that early weaning from PN and the use of PN cycling are protective factors; while LE (2010) states that the first and most effective therapeutic measure for a patient with PNALD is to minimise (if possible withdraw) PN followed by the introduction of enteral/oral nutrition. In most cases where the intensity of this pathology is mild to moderate, the measures described above (early use of enteral feeding, use of cycles of PN) solve the problem (VILLARES, 2008).

Finally, Borges et al. (2011) state that "due to the significant rate of complications observed with the prolonged use of PN, as well as its high cost, every effort should be made to maximise the use of oral and enteral nutrition".

4A.2.2 Enteral/oral nutrition

Although many patients with intestinal failure due to CIS require PN for survival, enteral feeding, when possible, should be started as soon as possible. Compared to NP, NE is more physiological (which makes it an excellent choice for accelerating intestinal adaptation and rehabilitation), safer and more economical (LE et al., 2010).

It is interesting to realise that the absorption capacity and, consequently, the tolerability of NE fluctuates depending on the degree of adaptation of the remaining intestine. Knowing that intestinal length is a very important contributing factor in adaptation, it is understood that patients who have at least ten centimetres of terminal ileum, preservation of the ileocecal valve and an intact ascending colon are unlikely to develop severe malnutrition or require greater nutritional support (NIGHTINGALE J.; WOODWARD M., 2006).

In simplistic terms, a diet rich in complex carbohydrates and low in fat is the goal. The transition from parenteral to enteral diet should be slow and gradual, not abandoning the PN prematurely. A good proportion of calories/day would be: 60 per cent carbohydrates, 20 per cent proteins and no more than 30g of fats (DANI, 2006). This aforementioned diet reflects the ideal for patients with an intact colon. Simple sugars such as fruit juices should be limited because they increase the osmotic load in the gastrointestinal tract and exacerbate diarrhoea (PAREKH, N.; SEIDNER D.; STEIGER E., 2005).

Patients with CIS (compromised terminal ileum and colon) have great impairment in the absorption of long-chain fatty acids, and their consumption is associated with worsening diarrhoea. In theory, the ideal diet for short bowel patients should contain the minimum amount of lipids, but in practice this is practically impossible. This hypothetical low-fat diet, despite increasing the absorption of calcium, magnesium and zinc, would leave the body's fatty acid reserves depleted. Finally, a good alternative source of energy would be the consumption of medium-chain triglycerides, as in addition to vitally reducing the incidence of nephrolithiasis, they have good absorption throughout the intestine (PAREKH, N.; SEIDNER D.; STEIGER E., 2005).

Among those who cannot tolerate the transition from NP to oral nutrition, Gong et al. (2009) suggest tube feeding; this helps the adaptive process and enhances absorptive capacity.

Short bowel sufferers should be encouraged to eat much more than usual to compensate for malabsorption. They should consume small portions throughout the day, rather than at set times. For those with colon continuity, in addition to a diet rich in complex carbohydrates containing starch, the diet should contain non-starch polysaccharides and soluble fibre. Studies have indicated that up to 525-1170 kcals per day can be absorbed provided you have an intact colon. The amount of energy absorbed is proportional to the length of the residual colon and may increase as part of the adaptive response to enterectomy (SEETHARAM, P.; RODRIGUES G., 2011).

Patients with limited ileal resection (less than 100 cm) with or without right hemi-colectomy can resume eating solid food in the late post-operative phase. These patients can develop diarrhoea or steatorrhoea with the consumption of a regular diet, due to fat malabsorption, which in turn can lead to deficiencies of fat-soluble vitamins, vitamin B12, calcium and magnesium. Deficiencies of these nutrients should always be investigated and supplemented if necessary (SEETHARAM, P.; RODRIGUES G., 2011).

Micronutrient supplementation should be individualised. According to Sundaram (2002 apud GARCIA, M.M.; MENENDEZ-CONDE, C.P.; VICEDO, T.B, 2011), lipid- and water-soluble vitamins should be supplemented. Vitamin D should be supplemented at a dose of 50000 IU; in patients who have had ileal resection greater than 60 cm, vitamin B12 will be replenished daily until 1000 mcg per month is reached. The other vitamins will have their plasma levels maintained with the use of multivitamins (GARCIA, M.M.; MENENDEZ-CONDE, C.P.; VICEDO, T.B, 2011).

Certain precautions must be taken with the diet in order to reduce some of the complications inherent in CIS. In order to avoid, for example, the formation of kidney stones, in addition to the precautions already mentioned regarding the intake of long-chain fatty acids, care must be taken to avoid dehydration; reducing the intake of oxalate is essential, avoiding the consumption of spinach, beetroot, nuts, chocolate, tea, wheat bran and strawberries (DIBIASE, J.K; YOUNG, R.J; VANDE- RHOOF, J.A., 2004).

Despite all the appropriate measures for good oral/enteral nutrition, patients who persist in losing weight and who do not absorb more than 30 per cent of the diet offered should use PN (PAREKH, N.; SEIDNER D.; STEIGER E., 2005).

4.4.3 Drug management

After a sudden loss of digestive capacity due to a massive resection, it is known

that structural and functional changes occur in the remaining intestine in an attempt to compensate, known as intestinal adaptation. If this adaptive response is insufficient, intestinal failure due to CIS occurs. Various hormones and drugs have been studied as potential enhancers of the intestinal adaptive process. Glutamine, growth hormone (GH), insulin-like growth factor (IGF-1), epidermal growth factor (EGF) and glucagon-like peptide (GLP-2) are the main substances that have been shown to potentiate the intestinal adaptive process.
currently being studied in terms of their trophic effect on the intestinal mucosa (MCMELLEN etal., 2010).

There have been several studies in animal models, until, little by little, in recent years, growth hormone has been gaining ground in human clinical trials. Although the use of GH in CIS has limited and conflicting results, based on preliminary animal studies, exogenous GH stimulates structural and functional adaptation of the intestine; it significantly increases the growth of the small intestinal mucosa, causing an increase in the absorption of liquids, electrolytes and nutrients. Some adverse effects of GH use have been observed, such as peripheral oedema and carpal tunnel syndrome (paresthesia and weakness in the hand) (WALES, 2010).

A promising observation made by McMellen et al. (2010) is that GH, due to its known trophic effect, can produce an increase in intestinal length; this becomes especially important when considering that the size of the remaining intestine is the biggest determinant of whether or not long-term use of NP is necessary.

Research, which is scarce at the moment, shows that GH, in low doses, associated or not with glutamine, is a potential short-term therapeutic modality for newly-resected patients; however, the real benefit of this treatment over time is not known. Therefore, there is insufficient evidence to determine the ideal duration of treatment and long-term safety (WALES, 2010).

Glutamine is an essential precursor substrate in nucleotide biosynthesis. It has been extensively studied in the treatment of CIS; its metabolic effects in the small intestine are well known (MIRANDA et al., 2006). Wales (2010) comments that glutamine is often used alone or in combination with growth hormone, which, in animal models, has a synergistic effect on the gastrointestinal tract, causing short-term weight gain due to increases in nutrient absorption; however, this effect is not observed when treatment is discontinued. Further studies are also needed to prove its true benefits.

EGF (epidermal growth factor) has been shown to be important for healing gastric ulcers and maintaining the normal architecture of the intestine. Mcmellen et al. (2010) demonstrated that the use of EGF promotes an increase in intestinal length in animals that had 50% of their intestines dried out; at a cellular level, it stimulates the synthesis of messenger RNA, DNA and proteins; at a histological level, it increases the height of the villi and the depth of the intestinal crypts. In this same study, the efficacy of EGF administration was only demonstrated if it was administered immediately after resection, which indicates that this substance only acts during the period when the intestine is in the process of adaptation, and thus has no effect when this adaptation reaches a plateau.

Several studies have shown that the use of GLP-2 (involved in regulating motility, intestinal permeability as well as crypt cell proliferation and nutrient absorption) implies hypertrophy and increased intestinal weight; it has also been shown to increase blood flow to the intestine and the activity of specific glucose transport proteins such as GLUT-2 (MARTIN et al., 2004).

An analogue of GLP-2, teduglutide, which is also related to restoring the structural and functional integrity of the intestine, promotes mucosal growth, reducing gastric emptying and secretion, thus leading to greater absorption of nutrients in patients with CIS. (JEPPESEN et al., 2011).

At doses ranging from 0.05 to 0.10 mg/kg/day of teduglutide, Jeppesen et al. (2011), in a partially closed study, showed that it was possible to reduce the dependence on PN in patients with short bowel; however, the study warns that more research will be needed to determine whether this reduction in the volume of parenteral feeding will also imply a reduction in complications and an improvement in quality of life. It was also observed that the beneficial effects of using teduglutide were reversible three weeks after its suspension, which suggests that chronic use of this drug may be necessary in patients with CIS.

Insulin-like growth factor (IGF-1), like GH, has been implicated in improving the proliferation capacity of post-resected enterocytes. It is postulated that IGF-1 is a mediator or even a permissor of GH action. In animal models, IGF-1 enabled weaning from PN. There are still no clinical trials on the action of IGF-1 in humans with short intestines (MCMELLEN etal., 2010).

4.5 Surgical Management

We have already commented in this same paper that the most important aspect that should remain in the mind of the surgeon who manages patients with a potential chance of developing CIS, such as patients with mesenteric infarction and Crohn's disease, is resection limited to the complications, thus trying to prevent intestinal failure due to short bowel. If necessary, reoperations need to be scheduled in order to more precisely delineate which bowel should really be resected and which should be kept.

The primary aim of surgical therapy is to increase the absorptive capacity of the intestine, either by transplantation or by techniques discussed later in this paper.

4.5.1 Bowel transplantation

A plausible approach for patients with intestinal insufficiency is to perform an organ transplant - IT (intestinal transplant). The indications for this type of treatment, while appealingly logical, are fraught with difficulties. The need for aggressive immunosuppression, rejection that is difficult to control, serious infections, a delicate surgical procedure, difficulties in preserving the graft, lymphoproliferative diseases, among others, limit the usual indication for IT (GALVÃO, 2003).

Since the 1960s, man has been endeavouring to develop intestinal transplants. The first successful case took place in Pittsburgh in 1980. By June 2008, there were more than 70 IT programmes worldwide. At the end of 2005, there were 1292 reported intestinal transplants (BUCKEL et al., 2009). The indication for IT is most commonly found in the child population - around 70 per cent of the total. This is a result of the difficulties and complications more frequently encountered in infants with regard to central access (used for PN), such as the occurrence of sepsis and troboembolic phenomena with the loss of this access; it has also been noted, as previously mentioned, that in children there is a higher incidence of metabolic disorders linked to PN. (GALVÃO, 2003).

Lao et al. (2010) state that there is a slight predominance of intestinal transplantation in males (57%); and that the pathology that most often leads patients to IT is gastroschisis (21%).

Candidates for IT can be categorised into patients with intestinal insufficiency only - they should receive an isolated intestinal transplant; patients with advanced PNALD - they should undergo liver transplantation in addition to intestinal transplantation; and finally, patients with multiple organ insufficiency who require multivisceral transplantation (GALVÃO, 2003).

A fourth transplant modality recently proposed by some researchers for patients with CIS is isolated liver transplantation (ILT). Spag- nuolo, M.I.; Ruberto, E.; Guarino, A. (2009) describes that TIF was initially performed on patients with short bowel movements as an emergency (these patients, due to prolonged use of NP, developed PNALD followed by liver failure) while awaiting intestinal grafting. In fact, it has been observed that patients who have a good expectation of intestinal adaptation and who develop liver failure have a higher survival rate if they receive TIF than those who receive combined liver and intestinal transplantation.

Dell'Olio et al. (2009 apud SPAGNUOLO, M.I.; RUBERTO, E.; GUARINO, A., 2009) suggest some criteria for TIF: 1- liver failure associated with established intestinal insufficiency (persistently high serum bilirubin, moderate/severe fibrosis, portal hypertension); 2- presence of at least 50 cm of functioning small intestine (without VIC) or 30 cm with VIC; 3- tolerated oral intake of at least 50 per cent of the estimated energy requirement, associated with weight gain, for four weeks before developing liver disease. It goes without saying that the length and functionality of the intestinal remnant is important for the success of TIF.

Patients who develop liver failure due to prolonged use of NP and who have an irreversible condition of intestinal failure (insufficient intestinal length, ineffective adaptation, etc.) are candidates for combined liver and intestinal transplantation. Galvão (2003) argues that this type of transplant accounts for half of all transplants in patients with CIS. Despite a low survival rate, combined intestine/liver transplantation is associated with better survival of the intestinal graft and a lower incidence of rejection compared to isolated intestinal transplants (SPAGNUOLO, M.I.; RUBERTO, E.; GUARINO, A., 2009).

> In multivisceral transplantation, several abdominal viscera are transplanted en bloc. It is indicated in cases of multiple abdominal organ failure due to severe dysmotility of the gastrointestinal tract, occlusion of the celiac trunk, thrombosis of the mesenteric-portal venous system or extensive polyposis of the digestive tract (GALVÃO, 2003, p. 120).

According to Pironi et al. (2010), when and which patients are candidates for IT is still a matter of great controversy and discussion; however, in an attempt to facilitate the management of patients with CIS, Gupte et al. (2006) suggested a list of indications and contraindications for intestinal transplantation (Table 3).

Table 3 - Indications and contraindications for intestinal transplantation

INDICATIONS	ABSOLUTE CONTRAINDICATIONS
<ul><li>Imperative need for NP with venous access impossible</li><li>Progressing liver disease with coagulopathy</li><li>Ascites and encephalopathy</li><li>Risk of death from sepsis associated with the catheter</li></ul>	<ul><li>Profound neurological impairment</li><li>Life-threatening diseases not related to the gastrointestinal tract</li><li>Non-resectable malignant tumours</li></ul>**RELATIVE**<ul><li>Immune deficiency (congenital or acquired)</li><li>Autoimmune disease</li><li>Insufficient vascular permeability to guarantee access for up to six months after transplantation</li><li>Chronic lung disease (in premature infants)</li></ul>

Source: (GUPTE et al., 2006, p. 262).

Graft rejection remains the biggest challenge to intestinal transplantation; in the short term, rejection affects up to 85 per cent of those transplanted, with graft loss estimated at 20 per cent (BUCKEL et al., 2009).

As it is an organ rich in lymphoid tissue and therefore has a high anti-genetic potential, immunosuppression is a key step in the success of IT; with greater knowledge and development of immunosuppressants, survival rates have reached 80% and 63% in one and five years, respectively (BUCKEL et al., 2009; LEE et al., 2002).

The appearance of the immunosuppressant Tacrolimus (FK-506) was a major breakthrough for the clinical success of intestinal transplants. FK-506 soon became the immunosuppressant of choice in IT; its use showed a longer survival with a greater chance of the graft functioning well, it caused fewer side effects and, above all, it controlled rejection more effectively (GALVÃO, 2003).

The initial post-IT phase requires intense clinical and laboratory monitoring; high doses of immunosuppressants are necessary to avoid rejection. Renal dysfunction, hypertension, neuropsychic problems and favourable infections, especially opportunistic ones, are common adverse effects of immunosuppressants (GALVÃO, 2003).

Intense immunosuppression, as previously discussed, predisposes the patient to sepsis due to opportunistic infections, especially CMW (BUCKEL et al., 2009); hence the preference for donors who have negative serology for CMV (except when the transplant is urgent). (GALVÃO, 2003).

It is extremely difficult to establish an early diagnosis of intestinal graft rejection, but it is of fundamental importance, because recognising this biological phenomenon as soon as possible makes it possible to reverse the condition with the appropriate use of immunosuppressants before the graft is lost. Given the lack of specific serological markers and the non-specificity of the clinical picture, the only alternative for establishing the diagnosis is a histopathological study using biopsies (diagnostic accuracy of around 60%) (LEE et al., 2004).

In a study carried out on animal models, Lee et al. (2004) observed that from the fifth day post-transplant, in rats in which interleukin-6 and IFN-Y WERE detected, there was a good correlation (no better than histopathology) with graft rejection.

The ideal transplant or management of patients with CIS remains controversial. Spagnuolo, M.I.; Ruberto, E.; Guarino, A. (2009) advocate combined intestine/liver transplantation as the standard because it has a lower incidence of rejection (perhaps due to the immunological tolerance induced by the liver); however, they note that isolated liver transplantation (in correctly indicated patients) can supplant combined transplantation in both the short and long term. Pironi et al. (2010) advocate that, as long as the patient has central access and does not have significant liver disease, the main treatment for patients with CIS is NP. Finally, among those who argue in favour of IT over NP, Galvão (2003) highlights the costs of both procedures: it is estimated that the costs of home NP are around US$120,000/year, while the costs of isolated intestinal, combined liver and multivisceral transplants have been falling over five years and are around US$132,285; US$214,716 and US$219,098; respectively, thus demonstrating the greater financial viability of IT over NP.

4.5.2 Surgical techniques (without transplantation)

Although intestinal transplantation has evolved, this technique remains little used due to various factors such as technical difficulty and availability in only a few centres around the world (OGAZÓN, 2008). So-called 'no-transplant' surgeries are used to treat CIS and fulfil at least one of these conditions: prolonging the transit of the intestine or increasing the absorption surface of the intestine (SEETHARAM, P.; RODRIGUES G., 2011).

Various techniques have been tried over the years in animal models or even in humans, however, we will highlight some of these imminently practical and promising surgical modalities from a therapeutic point of view: the Biachi technique, serial transverse enteroplasty (STEP), multiple colonic anastomoses, intestinal segment inversion and intestinal neomucosa implantation. The first two lend themselves to promoting intestinal lengthening and improving intestinal adaptation; they have high complication and failure rates, but are options that offer less complexity and lower risks than transplantation (FRANZON et al., 2010).

Undoubtedly the most widely used non-transplant surgical technique is the Bianchi technique. This technique, described by Bianchi in 1980, aims to increase the length of the remaining intestine. It consists of a longitudinal dissection, about 5cm from the mesenteric border, then a longitudinal division of the intestine, dividing it into two halves with half the diameter (preserving its vascularisation) and then anastomosing (end-to-end), doubling its previous length. It is recommended that the candidate for this procedure be at least 3 cm in diameter and 40 cm in intestinal length (BELLOLIO et al., 2010).

Perhaps the biggest obstacle to the Bianchi procedure is the need for an experienced surgeon. Technical difficulties include the risk of intense bleeding due to mesenteric vascular injury and the numerous sutures along the intestinal tract (OGAZÓN et al., 2008).

By increasing the final length of the intestine, this technique allows patients to tolerate more oral food content and in some cases (according to some reports) become NP-independent (OGAZÓN et al., 2008).

STEP (serial transverse enteroplasty) is summarised as a series of partial transverse sections along the intestine, establishing a zigzag-shaped channel that reduces the lumen but increases the intestinal length (Figure 2). It is indicated for those who are refractory to clinical treatment (BELLOLIO et al., 2010).

Technically easier to perform because there are no anastomoses (the intestine is not opened, nor is the mesentery altered), STEP can overcome the technical limitations of the Bianchi procedure. The technique is safer when applied with a linear stapler perpendicular to the longitudinal axis of the small intestine. STEP allows for an improvement in absorptive capacity and therefore better nutrition and weight maintenance (FRANZON et al., 2010).

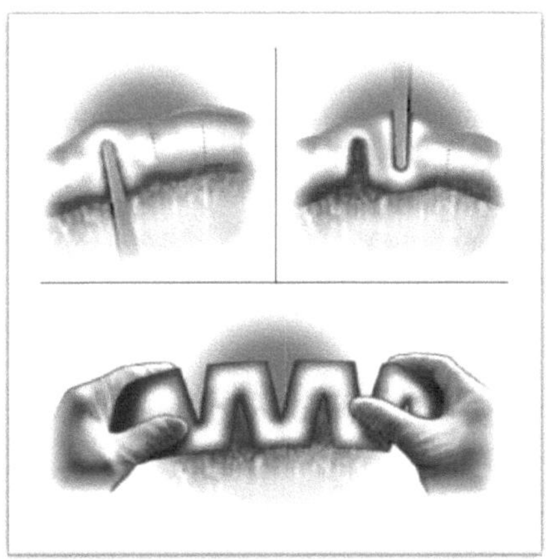

Figure 2 Serial transverse enteroplasty (STEP)
SOURCE: Bellolio et al. (2010, p. 479).

Ogazón et al. (2008) present another technique that can be used in CIS. Because it is simple, the technique of multiple colonic anastomoses offers less skilled surgeons and less specialised surgical centres the possibility of control and palliative treatment in intestinal insufficiency.

> First step: the abdominal cavity is approached, [...] the primary objective is to identify the proximal portion of the jejunum and the distal portion of the colon. [...] Second step: the stump of the left colon is cut. In two suture planes, an end-to-side anastomosis is made in one of the planes between the proximal jejunum and the transverse colon. The colon is then sectioned at the rectosigmoid junction. Third step: the sigmoid is anastomosed end-to-side with the transverse colon and the rectal stump is anastomosed with the left colon in the same way (Figure 3) (OGAZÓN et al., 2008, p. 44).

With this procedure, greater hydroelectrolytic control is possible, as well as greater control of amino acid, lipid and fluid requirements. The great enthusiasm for this surgical modality is the real gain in quality of life for patients undergoing it: after the procedure, they tolerate consuming a light diet (an opportunity for them to savour their food), greater control of their bowel habits and, because they require less intravenous nutritional demand, PN can be administered only at night, which gives them the day off to carry out normal daily activities (OGAZÓN et al., 2008).

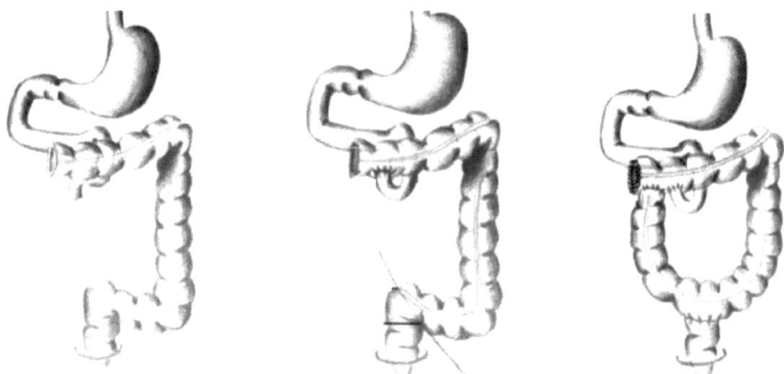

Figure 3 Multiple anastomosis technique in the colon.
SOURCE: Ogazón et al. (2008, p. 44-45).

In 1969, Rygick and Nasarov suggested a 20 cm ileal segment inversion technique, creating an anisoperistaltic mechanism[i] of the small intestine, slowing down the passage of chyme and increasing absorption. Long segments of intestine used in this technique produce obstructive conditions (Figure 4) (FRANZON et al., 2010).

A new approach to the treatment of CIS, which is still lacking studies, is the development of engineering for the construction of small intestine tissues.
Lloyd et al. (2006) explain the technique:

> The technique behind this concept is to employ an artificial biodegradable scaffold (in tubular form) to promote the growth of soft tissue tissues. Polylactic acid (PLA) and polyglycolic acid (PGA) have been used in small intestine tissue engineering in rodents as synthetic structures to support the adhesion and growth of "organelle units". These units consist of organelles from intestinal epithelial cells, stem cells, enterocytes and intestinal stromal cells. They are derived from neonatal intestinal tissue. [...] these units are placed in tubular scaffolds which are then immersed in the peritoneum of rodents (Lloyd et

---

[i] Peristalsis with contrary movement; antiperistalsis.

al., 2006, p. 27).

At the implant site, a kind of cystic structure is formed consisting of a surface with histological characteristics of the small intestine called "intestinal neomucosa". These neomucosa implants in rats develop and become functionally similar to normal intestinal mucosa. (FREUD, E; ESHET, R, 2001).

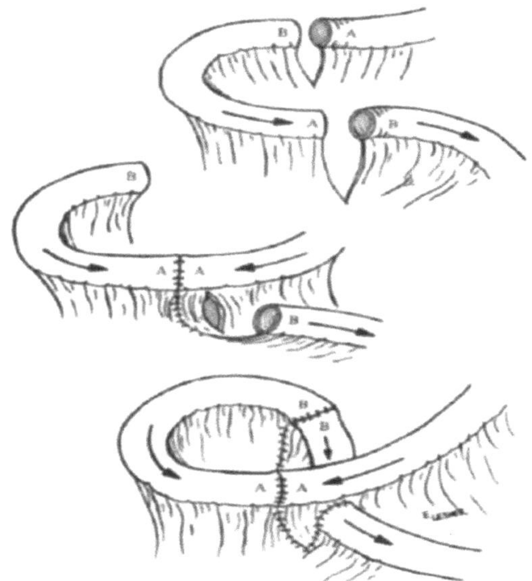

Figure 4 Rygick and Nasarov technique - making an anisoperistaltic loop segment.
SOURCE: Franzon et al. (2010, p. 53).

A major difficulty is still the need for many donors to make each neomucosa "cyst". Further work is needed to investigate new ways of improving the yield of the process and to identify other sources of donor tissue (LLOYD et al., 2006).

5 FINAL CONSIDERATIONS

It's clear that the subject discussed in this article has aroused the interest of countless researchers for many years. CIS encompasses controversies ranging from conceptual issues to its extremely varied prognosis.

The growing knowledge about the pathophysiology and the resulting adaptive processes of the intestine has, over the last few decades, led to vertiginous progress in the management of patients with CIS.

In this book, we realise that the drugs and measures commonly used in short- and long-term management, such as antidiarrhoeal drugs, octreotide (somatostatin analogue), proton pump inhibitors or anti-H2 inhibitors, trace element, vitamin and fluid replacement, are currently valid and should always form part of the foundation of the treatment of any patient with short bowel failure.

The nutrition of these patients continues to be one of the biggest challenges in this pathology. PN is essential for achieving higher survival rates; it is necessary at least in the first few weeks after surgery. The biggest determinant of its necessity, among other factors, is the length of the remaining intestine. NP has a number of limitations for its prolonged use: high cost, catheter-related infections leading to sepsis (in some situations), impaired intestinal adaptation and, on several occasions, liver failure. Although indispensable, NP should not be seen as a therapeutic end, but as a means, always aiming for oral nutrition.

In order to make the short intestine self-sufficient, stimulating its adaptation and promoting greater absorption capacity, various drugs such as GLP-2, GH, teduglutide, EGF, IGF-1 and glutamine have been studied, especially in animal models, showing promising results, but with limited scientific relevance.

In addition to drugs, excellence in intestinal transplantation has been sought for many years. With the introduction of more effective immunosuppressants such as Tacrolimus (FK-506), IT has gained new momentum in recent years. However, there are still high levels of graft rejection in transplant patients. The unavailability of IT in most of the world's medical centres makes this therapeutic modality very limited.

Given the difficulty of intestinal transplantation, surgeons all over the world are endeavouring to develop surgical techniques that try to prolong intestinal length or slow down intestinal transit. Some of these techniques deserve special mention because they are easier to perform and have shown relative success in reducing the need for PN or even completely rehabilitating patients with CIS. In this endeavour, the Bianchi technique and serial transverse enteroplasty (STEP) are the most widely used and most studied.

The scarcity of human studies does not allow us to pragmatise the ideal treatment for patients with CIS. This management should take into account the peculiarities of each case and the limitations of the medical centres and the healthcare team, thus arriving at a better, individualised and more efficient therapeutic choice ente.

REFERENCES

BANERJEE, A.; WARWICKER, P. Acute renal failure and metabolic disturbances in the short bowel syndrome. **Q. J. Med.,** Stevenage, United Kingdom, v. 95, p. 37-40, 2002. BELLOLIO, F.R. et al. Serial transverse enteroplasty as an alternative in the treatment of short bowel syndrome. Clinical case. **Rev. Med. Chile,** v. 138, p. 478-482, 2010.

BORGES, V.C. et al. Long-term nutritional assessment of patients with severe short bowel syndrome managed with home enteral nutrition and oral intake. **Nutrición Hospitalaria,** v. 26, n. 4, p. 834-42, 2011.

BUCKEL, E. et al. First intestinal transplant in Chile. Clinical case. **Rev. Méd. Chile,** v. 137, p. 259-263, 2009.

CASTILLO, C. et al. National experience in the management of short bowel syndrome in infants. **Rev. Chil. Paediatr.,** v.67, n. 3, p. 121-124, 1996.

CHAGAS NETO, F.A. et al. Intestinal transit examination in short bowel syndrome. **Radiol. Bras,** v. 44(3), p. 188-191, May/June 2011.

COLE, C.R. et al. Very Low Birth Weight Preterm Infants With Surgical Short Bowel Syndrome: Incidence, Morbidity and Mortality, and Growth Outcomes at18to 22 Months. **Pediatrics: Official Journal of the American Academy of Pediatrics,** v. 122, n. 3, Sep 2008.

. The rate of bloodstream infection is high in infants with short bowel syndrome: Relationship with small bowel bacterial overgrowth, enteral feeding and in- flammatory and immune responses. **Journal Pediatrics,** v. 156, n. 6, p. 941-947, Jun2010.

DANI, R. **Essential Gastroenterology.** 3. ed. Rio de Janeiro: Guanabara Koogan, 2006.

DIBIASE, J.K; YOUNG, R.J; VANDERHOOF, J.A. Intestinal Rehabilitation and the Short Bowel Syndrome: Part 1. **American Journal Gastroenterologv,** v. 99, p. 1386-95, 2004.

. Intestinal Rehabilitation and the Short Bowel Syndrome: Part 1. American Journal Gastroenterology, v. 99, P. 1823-1832, 2004.

DROZDOWSKI, L., THOMSON, A.B.R. Intestinal mucosal adaptation. **World Journal Gastroenterol,** v. 12, n. 29, p. 4614-4627, Aug 2006.

DURAN, B. The effects of long-term total parenteral nutrition on gut mucosal immun- ity in children with short bowel syndrome: a systematic review. **BMC Nurs.,** v. 4,n.1, Feb 2005.

FRANZON, O. et al. Short bowel syndrome: a new alternative for surgical treatment. **ABCD Arq. Bras. Cir. Dig.;** São José, SC, Brazil, v 23, n 1,p 51-55, 2010.

FREUD, E; ESHET, R. Insightsfrom animal modelsforgrowing intestinal neomucosa with serosal patching - a still untapped technique for the treatment of short bowel syndrome. **LaboratoryAnimals Ltd. LaboratoryAnimals,** Tel Aviv, Israel, v. 35, p. 180-187, 2001.

GALVÃO, F.H.F. Degated Intestine Transplantation. **Arq. Gastroenterol.,** v. 40, n. 2, Apr/Jun 2003.

GARCIA, M.M.; MENENDEZ-CONDE, C.P.; VICEDO, T.B. Advances in the knowledge of the use of micronutrients in artificial nutrition. **Nutrición Hospitalaria,** v. 26, n.1, p. 37-47, 2011.

GIL, A. C. **Como elaborar projetos de pesquisa.** 4. ed. São Paulo; Atlas, 2002.

GONG, J.F. et al. Role ofenteral nutrition in adult short bowel syndrome undergoing intestinal rehabilitation: the long-term outcome. **Asia Pac. J. Clin. Nutr.,** v. 18, n. 2, p. 155-16, 2009.

GUPTE, G.L. et al. Current issues in the management of intestinal failure. **Arch. Dis. Child,** Birmingham, United Kingdom, v. 91, p. 259-264, 2006.

GURA, K. M. et al. Reversal of Parenteral Nutrition-Associated Liver Disease in Two Infants With Short Bowel Syndrome Using Parenteral Fish Oil: Implications for Future Management. **Pediatrics: Official Journal of the American Academy of Pediatrics,** v. 118,n. 1,Jul 2006.

. Safety and Efficacy of a Fish-Oil-Based Fat Emulsion in the Treatment of Parenteral Nutrition-Associated Liver Disease. **Pediatrics: Official Journal of the American Academy of Pediatrics,** v. 121, n. 3, p. 678-86, Mar2008.

HASOSAH, M. et al. Congenital short bowel syndrome: A case report and review of the literature. **Can. Journal Gastroenterology,** v. 22 ,n. 1, p. 71-74, 2008.

JEPPESEN, P.B. Clinicai Significance ofGLP-2 in Short-Bowel Syndromel. **Journal of Nutrition,** Copenhagen, Denmark, v. 133, p. 3724-3724, 2003.

. Randomised placebo-controlled trial ofteduglutide in reducing parenteral nu- trition and/or intravenous fluid requirements in patients with short bowel syndrome **Gut,** v. 60, p. 902-914, 2011.

JOLY, F. et al. Morphological adaptation with preserved proliferation/transporter content in the colon of patients with short bowel syndrome. **American Journal Physiology Gastrointest Liver Physiol.,** v 297, p. 116-123, Apr 2009.

LAO, O.B. et al. Outcomes in Children After Intestinal Transplant. **Pediatrics,** Seat- tle, Washington; v. 125, n. 3, p. 550-558, Mar2010.

LE, H.D. et al. Innovative Parenteral and Enteral Nutrition Therapy for Intestinal. **Semin. Paediatr. Surg.,** v.19,n.1, Feb2010.

LEE, A.D.W. et al. Study of Morbidity In Orthotopic Small Intestine Transplantation With Wistar Rats - Experimental Study. **Arq. Gastroenterol,** São Paulo, SP, Brazil, v. 39, n.1,p. 39-47, Jan/Mar2002.

. Involvement of cytokines in acute rejection of intestinal transplants in rats. **Arq. Gastroenterol.,** São Paulo, SP, Brazil, v. 41, n. 2, p. 114-120, Apr/Jun 2004.

LLOYD, D.A.J. et al. Pilot study investigating a novel subcutaneously implanted pre-cellularised scaffold fortissue engineering ofintestinal mucosa. **European Cells and Materials,** v.11,p. 27-34, 2006.
KEMP, R. et al. Liver disease associated with intestinal failure in the small bowel syndrome. **Acta Cirúrgica Brasileira,** v.21,n.1, p. 67-71,2006.

MARCONI, M.A.; LAKATOS, E.M. **Fundamentos de metodologia científica.** 6. ed.- São Paulo: Atlas, 2005.

MARTINEZ, M. et al. Evolución y sobrevida de pacientes pediátricos con Síndrome de Intestino Corto (SIC). **Nutrition and Diet Therapy Department. Hospital de Ninos "SorMaría Ludovica",** Buenos Aires, Argentina, v. 26, n. 1,p. 239-242, 2011.
MARTIN, G.R. et al. Glucagon-like peptide-2 induces intestinal adaptation in parenterally fed rats with short bowel syndrome. **American Journal Physiology - Gastrointestinal Liver Physiology,** v. 286, p. 964-972, Feb 2004.

MCMELLEN, M.E. et al. Growth Factors: Possible Roles for Clinicai Management of the Short Bowel Syndrome. **Semin. Pediatr. Surg.,** v.19,n1,p. 35-43, Feb 2010.

MIRANDA, A.C. et al. Massive Intestinal Resection in Rats Fed up on Glutamine: hepatic glycogen content valuation. **Arq. Gastroenterol.,** v. 43, n. 1, Jan/Mar 2006.

MIRANDA, S.C. et al. Hypomagnesemia in short bowel syndrome patients. **J/Rev. Paul. Med.,** São Paulo, v. 118, n. 6, p. 169-72, 2000.

NIGHTINGALE J.; WOODWARD M. Guidelines for management of patients with a short bowel. **Gut;** v. 55 (Suppl IV), p 1-12, 2006

NONINO, C.B. et al. Oral Nutritional Therapy in Patients with Short Bowel Syndrome, **Rev. Nutr., Campinas,** v. 14, n. 3, p. 201-205, Sep/Dec, 2001.

OGAZÓN, F.R. et al. Multiple colonic anastomosis in the surgical treatment of the small intestine. A new technique. **Cir. Ciruj.** México, v. 76, p. 43-47, Jan/Feb 2008.

PALLE, L.; REDDY, B. Case report: Congenital short bowel syndrome. **Indian J. Radiol. Imaging,** v. 20, n. 3, p. 227-229, Aug 2010.

PAREKH, N.; SEIDNER D.; STEIGER E. Managing short bowel syndrome: Making the most of what the patient still has. **Cleveland Clinic Journal of Medicine,** v. 72, n 9, Sep 2005.

PENNINGTON, C.R. et al. Management of the short bowel syndrome. **SAJCN,** Dundee, Scotland v. 16, n. 2, Jul 2003.

PIRONI, L. et al. Long-term follow-up of patients on home parenteral nutrition in Europe: implications for intestinal transplantation. **Gut 2011,** Bologna, Italy; v. 60, p. 1725, 2010.

SAFIOLEAS, M. et al. Short Bowel Syndrome: Amelioration of Diarrhea afterVagot- omy and Pyloroplastyfor Peptic Haemorrhage. **Tohoku J. Exp. Med.,** v. 214, p. 7-10, 2008.
SEETHARAM, P.; RODRIGUES G. Short Bowel Syndrome: A Rewiew of Management Options. **Saudi J. Gastroenterol.,** Manipal, India, v.17, n. 4, p. 229-35, Jul/Aug, 2011.

SEVERINO, A.J. **Metodologia do trabalho científico.** 23. ed. São Paulo: Cortez, 2007.

SPAGNUOLO, M.I.; RUBERTO, E.; GUARINO, A. Isolated liver transplantation for treatment of liver failure secondary to intestinal failure. **Italian Journal of Paediatrics,** Napoli, Italy, v. 35, n. 28, Sep2009.

SPENCER, A.U. et al. Paediatric Short Bowel Syndrome Outcomes. **Annals of Sur-**

gery, Ohio, v. 242, n. 3, Sep 2005.

Paediatric short-bowel syndrome: the cost of comprehensive care. **American Journal of Clinical Nutrition,** v. 88, p. 1552-9, 2008.

TANNURI, U. Short bowel syndrome in children - treatment with home parenteral nutrition. **Rev Assoe Med Bras,** v. 50, n. 3, p. 330-7, 2004.

TOWSEND, C.M. et al. **Sabiston:** treatise on surgery. 17. ed. Rio de Janeiro: Elsevier, 2005.

VILLARES, J.M.M. Complicaciones hepáticas asociadas al uso de nutrición parente- ral. **Nutrición Hospitalaria,** v. 23 (Supl. 2), p. 25-33, 2008.

UNAMUNO, M.R.D.L. et al. Use of totally implanted venous catheters for parenteral nutrition: care, length of stay and occurrence of infectious complications. **Rev. Nutr., Campinas,** v. 18, n. 2, p. 261-269, Mar/Apr, 2005.

WALES, W.P. Human growth hormone and glutamine for patients with short bowel syndrome. **Cochrane Database of Systematic Reviews** Issue 6. Art. No.: CD006321.2010.

WANG, L. et al. Chronically administered retinoic acid has trophic effects in the rat small intestine and promotes adaptation in a resection model of short bowel syndrome. **American Journal Physiol. Gastrointest. Liver Physiol.,** v. 292, p. 15591569, 2007. WU, G.H. et al. Effects of bowel rehabilitation and combined trophic therapy on intestinal adaptation in short bowel patients. **World Journal Gastroenterol,** v.9,n.11, p. 2601-2604, 2003.

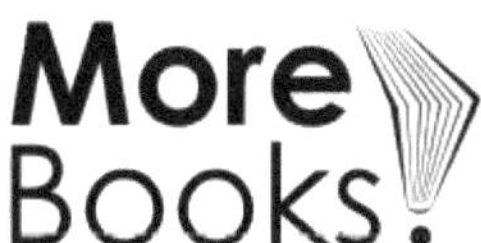

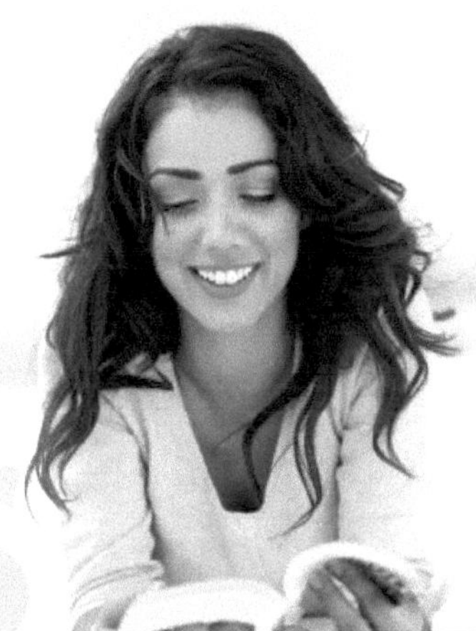

I want morebooks!

Buy your books fast and straightforward online - at one of world's fastest growing online book stores! Environmentally sound due to Print-on-Demand technologies.

Buy your books online at
www.morebooks.shop

Kaufen Sie Ihre Bücher schnell und unkompliziert online – auf einer der am schnellsten wachsenden Buchhandelsplattformen weltweit! Dank Print-On-Demand umwelt- und ressourcenschonend produzi ert.

Bücher schneller online kaufen
www.morebooks.shop

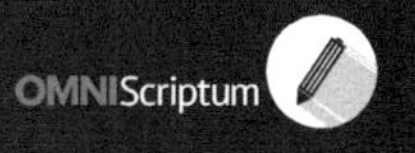

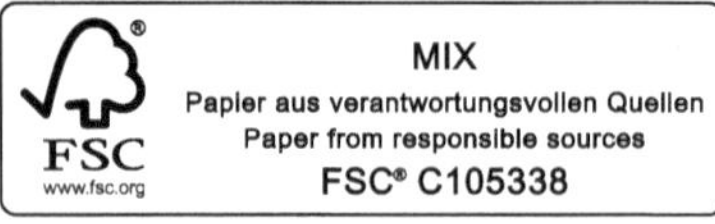

Printed by Books on Demand GmbH, Norderstedt / Germany